# MINDFULLY ATTACHED:

## Turning Out To Be Safer Throughout Everyday Life And Love

## By

## Carla C. Williams

# TABLE OF CONTENTS

# INTRODUCTION

In the many-sided embroidery of human connections, there exists a significant and wonderful idea known as "Mindfully Attached." This term embodies the substance of close to home association, the sensitive specialty of sustaining bonds, and the unflinching obligation to understanding and supporting each other. At its center, being mindfully connected in a relationship implies something beyond being together; it's about the profundity of presence, the delicacy of care, and the rugged string that ties central cores. Go along with me on an excursion through the charming domain of mindfully connected connections, where sympathy, compassion, and steadfast dedication make a romantic tale worth loving.

# CHAPTER 1

## The role of relationships

Connections are perplexing and diverse, and understanding the roles that each accomplice plays in a relationship is fundamental for keeping a solid and satisfying organization. Whether you are in a close connection or a kinship, understanding relationship roles is pivotal for making common regard and congruity between accomplices.

### Figuring out Relationship roles : What You Want to Be Aware

Connections are complicated and complex, and understanding the roles that each accomplice plays in a relationship is fundamental for keeping a sound and satisfying organization. Whether you are in a heartfelt connection or a kinship, understanding relationship roles is pivotal for making shared regard and congruity between accomplices.

## The Significance of Characterizing Relationship roles

Characterizing relationship roles explains each accomplice's liabilities and assumptions. It assists with taking out errors, clashes, and hatred between accomplices. At the point when each accomplice grasps their role in the relationship and consents to do their obligations, it prompts a more durable, fulfilling, and satisfying organization.

Furthermore, characterizing relationship roles can likewise assist with laying out limits and advance solid correspondence. By plainly characterizing what each accomplice is answerable for, it can keep one accomplice from feeling overpowered or troubled with assignments that they didn't consent to. It likewise considers transparent correspondence about any issues or worries that might emerge in the relationship, as each accomplice realizes what is generally anticipated of them and can resolve any issues in a valuable way.

## Orientation Generalizations and Relationship roles

## MINDFULLY ATTACHED

Orientation generalizations have mainly assumed a critical part in forming relationship roles. Society has long advanced the possibility that men ought to be suppliers while ladies ought to be overseers. Be that as it may, connections are not static and have developed over the long run, with additional individuals embracing sexually unbiased roles. Couples can decide to characterize their relationship roles in the manner they see fit, paying little heed to orientation.
Regardless of the headway made in separating orientation generalizations, they actually continue in numerous parts of society, including connections. For instance, studies have indicated that ladies actually do most family tasks and childcare, in any event, when they work all day outside the home. This can make pressure and hatred in connections, as one accomplice might feel overburdened and underestimated.

Couples really must have transparent correspondence about their assumptions and requirements in a relationship. This can assist with guaranteeing that the two accomplices feel esteemed and regarded, and that relationship roles are characterized such that works for the two people. By testing orientation generalizations and embracing sexually unbiased roles, couples can make more fair and satisfying connections.

## The Advancement of Relationship roles over the long run

Relationship roles have gone through massive changes throughout the long term. Customarily, men have been the essential providers, while ladies have been liable for dealing with the home and bringing up youngsters. In any case, the ascent of ladies' freedom developments and the changing monetary scene have prompted a change in relationship roles. These days, couples are bound to share liabilities similarly and focus on individual satisfaction.Besides, the idea of contemporary connections has become all the more broadly acknowledged as of late. Same-sex couples, polyamorous connections, and open connections are currently perceived and regarded by numerous social orders. This has prompted a more noteworthy comprehension and acknowledgment of different relationship roles and elements.

## The Various Sorts of Relationship roles

Relationship roles come in various structures, from customary orientation roles to forward-thinking orientation roles, to totally individualized roles. A few couples like to characterize their relationship roles by conventional orientation standards, while others decide to split away from those standards through and through and make their own novel roles. No matter what the kind of relationship role, the key is for the two accomplices to be in arrangement.

It is critical to take note that relationship roles can likewise change over the long run. As couples develop and advance, their necessities and assumptions might move, prompting a reexamination of their roles inside the relationship. This can be a sound and essential interaction, as it permits the two accomplices to convey their requirements and wants and make changes on a case by case basis. Couples must consistently check in with one another and have transparent discussions about their relationship roles to guarantee that the two accomplices feel appreciated and esteemed.

## Step-by-step instructions to Impart Successfully About Relationship roles

Compelling correspondence is fundamental for characterizing relationship roles. The two accomplices should be clear about their assumptions and necessities, and in settlement on how their obligations will be isolated. Legit and open correspondence will assist with forestalling false impressions and guarantee that the two accomplices feel appreciated and comprehended. It is additionally fundamental to routinely reconsider relationship roles and make changes as the need might arise.One compelling method for conveying about relationship roles is to plan customary registrations with your accomplice. This can be an assigned time every week or month when you both plunk down and examine how things are going concerning your roles and obligations. During these registrations, it's critical to listen effectively to your accomplice's interests and needs, and to communicate your own in a non-significant manner. By routinely checking in and imparting transparently, you can keep away from disdain and guarantee that the two accomplices feel esteemed and upheld in their roles.

## Grasping the Upsides and downsides of Conventional Orientation roles

Conventional orientation roles have been both applauded and reprimanded after some time. From one perspective, conventional orientation roles can give a reasonable division of obligations and a feeling of steadiness. Then again, they can likewise be restricting and keep the two accomplices from genuinely understanding their true capacity.

Understanding the upsides and downsides of customary orientation roles can assist couples with pursuing more educated choices while characterizing their relationship roles.

One of the primary benefits of conventional orientation roles is that they can give a feeling of commonality and solace. Many individuals grew up with guardians or grandparents who stuck to conventional orientation roles, and thus, they might feel more great and secure in connections that follow these equivalent examples. Furthermore, customary orientation roles can assist with laying out a feeling of request and construction inside a family, which can be useful for couples who esteem routine and consistency.Be that as it may, there are likewise a few disadvantages to customary orientation roles. For instance, they can build up unsafe generalizations and cutoff people's chances for individual and expert development. Ladies, specifically, might be supposed to focus on homegrown obligations over their professions, which can prompt sensations of disappointment and unfulfillment. Furthermore, customary orientation roles  can make power irregular characteristics inside connections, with one accomplice expecting a prevailing role and the other a compliant role.

## Factors That Impact Relationship roles

There are many elements that can impact relationship roles, including social, social, and financial variables. Social assumptions and normal practices can assume a critical part in forming what is viewed as proper conduct in a relationship. Monetary factors, for example, work plans and profound work can likewise affect relationship roles and division of obligations.Another element that can impact relationship roles is individual character attributes. For instance, somebody who is normally more decisive may take on an influential position in the relationship, while somebody who is more detached may take on a more steady role. Moreover, previous encounters and injuries can likewise influence how people approach and explore their roles in a relationship.

## The Effect of Culture on Relationship roles

Culture assumes a critical part in molding relationship roles. Various societies have various qualities and assumptions with regard to connections. In certain societies, it very well might be normal for ladies to take on conventional care taking roles, while in others, there might be more emphasis on individual satisfaction and fairness in connections.Besides, social standards can likewise impact the manner in which couples speak with one another. For instance, in certain societies, direct correspondence might be viewed as fierce or discourteous, while in others, it could be esteemed as a method for communicating genuineness and straightforwardness.

Moreover, social convictions about marriage and family can affect relationship roles. In certain societies, marriage is viewed as a joining between two families, rather than only two people. This can prompt more tension on couples to adjust to conventional orientation roles and family assumptions.

## Adjusting Fairness and Uniqueness in Connections

Making a solid and fulfilling organization implies finding some kind of harmony among equity and independence. Each accomplice ought to feel esteemed and regarded, and their remarkable necessities and wants ought to be thought of. It is fundamental to perceive that each accomplice will have their assets and shortcomings, and partitioning liabilities such that plays to those qualities and addresses any shortcomings is alright.

Notwithstanding, it is critical to abstain from falling into conventional orientation roles or accepting that specific errands or obligations are exclusively the obligation of one accomplice. Openness is of the utmost importance in guaranteeing that the two accomplices feel appreciated and comprehended, and that any lopsided characteristics or issues are tended to in a deferential and valuable way.One more significant part of adjusting equity and uniqueness in connections is keeping a feeling of freedom and independence. While it is normal to need to invest energy with your accomplice and pursue choices together, it is likewise essential to keep up with your advantages, leisure activities, and companionship. This considers self-improvement and satisfaction, yet additionally assists with forestalling codependency and disdain in the relationship.

## Procedures for Overseeing Clashes Over Relationship roles

In any event, when relationship roles are distinct, clashes can emerge. Various assumptions and errors can prompt conflicts and strain between accomplices. Methodologies for overseeing clashes in connections incorporate undivided attention, communicating needs obviously, and tracking down compromises that work for the two accomplices.Getting outside help, for example, couples advising, can likewise be a powerful method for exploring clashes in connections.

One significant procedure for overseeing clashes over relationship roles is to lay out clear limits and assumptions all along. This can assist with forestalling misconceptions and conflicts down the line. It's likewise vital to consistently check in with your accomplice and ensure that both of you are as yet OK with the roles you have laid out.Another successful methodology is to rehearse sympathy and attempt to see things according to your accomplice's viewpoint. This can assist you with figuring out their necessities and concerns, and track down arrangements that work for both of you. It's essential to move toward clashes with a receptive outlook and an eagerness to think twice about, then attempting to "win" the contention.

## Instructions to Make an Exceptional and Satisfying Organization Through Role Exploration

Exploring different relationship roles can prompt a seriously satisfying, remarkable organization. Exploring different avenues regarding various roles can assist couples with finding what turns out best for themselves and permits them to track down equilibrium and agreement in their relationship. It is vital to approach role exploration with a receptive outlook, convey sincerely and straightforwardly, and regard each other's necessities and wants.

All in all, understanding relationship roles is a significant piece of keeping a cheerful and satisfying organization. By exploring various kinds of relationship roles and straightforwardly conveying about assumptions, couples can make an extraordinary and amicable relationship that works for the two accomplices. Whether they decide to embrace customary orientation roles or select modern roles, the key is to move toward relationship roles with a receptive outlook, regard, and understanding.It is critical to take note that role exploration ought not be constrained or compelled upon one or the other accomplice. The two people ought to feel good and ready to try different things with various roles. It is additionally vital to consistently check in with each other and rethink the roles being investigated to guarantee that they are as yet working for the two accomplices. By moving toward role exploration with care and thought, couples can make major areas of strength for a satisfying organization that considers development and development over the long haul.

# CHAPTER 2

## What's the significance here To Have Restless Connection?

As per the connection hypothesis, you foster a connection style in youth that is affected by both hereditary elements and the connections you have with your guardians. As you progress in years, your connection style shapes how you explore cozy connections.There are four sorts of connection styles: secure, restless, avoidant, and muddled. In particular, individuals with restless connection styles long to feel near others yet battle to have a good sense of reassurance in their connections and dread being deserted by their loved ones.

### Indications of a Restless Connection Style

Having a restless connection style can influence how you act in a relationship, how you answer struggles, and how you feel about yourself. A trademark indication of a restless connection style is called hyperactivation, or continually searching for signs that your accomplice will leave you. This can seem to be:

1.Requiring incessant consolation (e.g., inquiring, "Do you actually cherish me?")
2.Fanatically searching for signs that your accomplice is pulling, ceaselessly
3.Seeing little issues as dangers to the whole relationship

Accepting the most obviously terrible about your accomplice's ways of behaving (e.g., expecting they haven't messaged you back since they couldn't care less about you, rather than thinking about different clarifications)

Different signs you could have a restless connection style include:
1.Having a negative perspective on yourself.
2.Ruminating over the most pessimistic scenario situations.
3.Continually agonizing over your relationship.
4.Needing to understand what your accomplice is thinking or feeling consistently.

While getting consolation or having a good second with an accomplice can offer impermanent help, these signals are many times sufficient not to encourage individuals with restless connection styles long haul. Eventually, somebody with a restless connection style struggles with believing their requirements will be met, and this nervousness can make them act in manners that appear to be doubtful or "tenacious."

## Causes

At the point when you're a kid, you depend on your parental figures for endurance. This incorporates your natural requirements (food, sanctuary, warmth) and feelings.Newborn children, for instance, will go to their essential parental figures when they are in trouble, like by crying when they're eager or looking for solace when they're apprehensive. How dependably their requirements are met at these times shapes how they come to see themselves as well as other people. As per the connection hypothesis, this is the way individuals create a "working model" of connection, which impacts how they view connections as grown-ups.At the point when guardians reliably meet both the physical and profound requirements of a youngster and provide their kid with a feeling of safety as they begin to investigate their environmental elements, that kid is bound to foster a protected connection style. At the point when a kid's necessities are met conflicting or not the slightest bit, that youngster is bound to foster an unreliable connection style, for example, restless, avoidant, or disordered connection.Youngsters with restless connection styles might have learned they need to perform flawlessness, carry on, or battle to keep their guardians close to get their requirements met. While these ways of behaving could have assisted them as kids, they become pointless in grown-up connections. Extra factors that can prompt the improvement of a restless connection style include:

1.Your parental figure's connection style.

2.Hereditary variables, for example, having a family background of nervousness.

3.Youth misuse (particularly from a guardian)

4.Losing a parent or one more guardian as a kid.

5.Life stressors that made your parental figure less accessible to you when you were youthful.

## What Can Set off Restless Connection?

For somebody with a restless connection style, their uneasiness might become uplifted in close connections. Occasions that can set off somebody with a restless connection style include:
1.Entering another close connection.
2.Distressing life altering situations.
3.Enormous relationship achievements (e.g., moving in together or getting hitched)
4.Struggle in the relationship.

While each relationship has some degree of contention, the stakes of these contentions could appear to be higher for somebody with a restless connection style. Clashes, contentions, or irregularities with your accomplice could set off a separation anxiety, making the individual with a restless connection style request consolation, stress over their accomplice leaving them, or earnestly need both physical or profound closeness to their cherished one.

## Impacts of a having a Restless Connection Style

Studies have shown that individuals with restless connection styles will generally report the accompanying:

1.More clash with their accomplices
2.Less confidence in their connections
3.A lower relationship fulfillment

These impacts could be a consequence of a restlessly connected individual's propensity to zero in on adverse occasions and expect the most terrible about their accomplice's goals. Hyperactivation ways of behaving, for example, having major areas of strength for a to a minor clash, can cause extra pressure in the relationship.Beyond connections, there are additional individual emotional well-being impacts that you could insight into assuming you have a restless connection. This incorporates being at a higher gamble of fostering some tension problems, misery, and low confidence.

## Step-by-step instructions to Adapt

It means quite a bit to take note of that while having restless connection can hear and there make connections troublesome, you're not ill-fated to be despondent seeing someone. As a matter of fact, concentrates to show that individuals with restless connection will generally show more appreciation in their connections and are in numerous instances exceptionally compassionate and on top of their accomplice's feelings.Assuming you think your restless connection style is influencing your connections, there are a few things you can attempt to assist with easing your concerns and feel more secure with your accomplice:

**Figure out your tension:** Recognizing your connection style and how it's connected with your life as a youngster encounters can assist with diminishing self-fault in connections. At the point when nervousness about your relationship creeps in, remind yourself this might be an injury from way back reemerging. Attempt to remain aware of your triggers and work on checking current realities before you have a response.

**Speak with your accomplice:** Let your accomplice in on what sets off your nervousness. Concoct a blueprint for exploring struggle and examine what you both need to make greater security in your relationship.

**Find approaches to self-manage your feelings:** Handling and directing your feelings with an accomplice can be a fundamental component of connections. Yet, for individuals with restless connection styles, it means quite a bit to track down ways of managing feelings all alone. This could seem to be giving yourself some space, paying attention to music, sprinkling cold water all over, rehearsing profound breathing methods, or going on a walk.

**Support your life beyond your relationship:** It very well may be not difficult to focus on your personal connections when you have a restless connection style. Yet, remember to keep up with your non-close connections as well.This could seem to be participating in exercises you appreciate without your accomplice, searching for help from companions, and investing energy with your loved ones.

## Fixing a Restless Connection Style

Your connection style can change after some time. Individuals with restless connection might start to feel more secure with a committed and secure accomplice who they've been with for a long time. This implies that it's conceivable the impacts of restless connection can turn out to be less obtrusive in long haul connections. Solid connections that incorporate clear correspondence and common regard can move your functioning model of connection, giving you new encounters that go against what you realized as a kid.

Furthermore, emotional well-being treatment can assist with supporting recuperation from a restless connection style whether you are in a heartfelt connection. The accompanying emotional wellness treatments have shown proof of assisting individuals with growing safer connection styles:

**Relational psychotherapy:** A kind of talk treatment that spotlights on further developing connections by dealing with troublesome responses, thought examples, and ways of behaving that happened in current or past connections.

**Mental conduct treatment:** A social treatment that spotlights on the connection between your viewpoints, feelings, and ways of behaving and moves pessimistic ideas examples and sentiments to assist with working on generally prosperity

**Psychodynamic treatment:** A discussion-based treatment that investigates the oblivious powers and youth encounters that influence your feelings and ways of behaving.

**Couples treatment:** Offers support for couples in serious relationships to assist with figuring out unambiguous triggers, work through relational struggles, and foster survival methods.

## The most effective method to Help Your Restlessly Connected Accomplice

Assuming you have an accomplice that has restless connection, it very well may be hard to tell how to best help them while likewise keeping up with your independence in the relationship. As well as looking for your help, here are far to help a collaborate with restless connection:

**Distinguish your connection style:** It tends to be useful to comprehend how your connection style appears in the relationship. For instance, on the off chance that you have an avoidant connection style, you may be additional delicate to your accomplice's requirement for closeness and make some harder memories meeting them midway.

**Practice clear and powerful correspondence:** Speak with your accomplice in an immediate and sympathetic way. For example, if you can't message your accomplice during the workday, discuss that with them, obviously. Try not to be obscure about your limits to forestall the chance of miscommunication and open doors for your accomplice to expect the most obviously terrible about the relationship.Individuals with restless connection styles battle to have a solid sense of reassurance in their connections. While they long to feel near their accomplices, this need is frequently determined by separation anxieties, questions, and low confidence. Your connection style creates in adolescence, however, can influence close connections as you age. Assuming you're restlessly appended, you might want to request consistent consolation, overanalyze your accomplice's ways of behaving, or have large responses to little contentions.

While restless connection can some time adversely influence your connections, fortunately safer connection can foster over the long haul. Tracking down a serious accomplice, figuring out how to impart your triggers, and looking for psychological wellness treatment are ways of expanding wellbeing in your connections, fostering a safer connection style, and lifting your confidence.

# CHAPTER 3

## The sacrificial Love

The idea of sacrificial love is a muddled one. To be really sacrificial, you need to put others first, and that occasionally implies settling on hard decisions.

I have battled for as long as I can remember with adoration. There are times when it seems like adoring somebody is narrow-minded, and afterward times when it is caring. The issue is that you can blur all through self-centered/magnanimous love as fast as you can flutter an eyelash. In some cases, it feels narrow-minded to need love, while different times you feel like you are the only one sacrificial in adoration. If it sounds confounding… it is.

The main way that I can characterize caring adoration is the point at which you are in it for the long stretch. Whether it harms, is difficult, or you don't receive anything in return for yourself, adoring somebody sacrificially implies that you pursue choices put together not regarding what you require, but rather what is best for the one you love.

## What does benevolent love resemble?

At the point when I was in my thirties, my better half was determined to have pancreatic disease. Out of nowhere, an organization that I consented to, transformed into a nursing relationship where I was liable for the children, the house, and him.Being sacrificial isn't generally so natural as it sounds. I recollect one day he got me on the telephone bitching about how he wasn't making a difference. How dare, he could scarcely get up! Yet, being caring isn't actually something people are best at.

All in all, what characterizes magnanimous love? Is it something to be thankful for or terrible? In one sense, it implies setting your requirements aside for later. Yet, on the off chance that there really is love, you need to forfeit yourself to get the best love of all. Do you need to forfeit every one of you? Not the least bit, but rather when the time calls for it, you do what you really want to do.

## Signs you're equipped for adoring selflessly

Do you believe you're a magnanimous, darling? Is it true that you are fit for cherishing somebody harming your joy? Here are the signs that put caring affection aside from narrow-minded love.

**You consideration more about the prosperity of somebody more than yourself:**There are times when benevolent love includes thinking often more about their prosperity than your own. That could imply that you accomplish something that isn't self-propelling because you realize that they truly need your assistance.Figuring out how to place others' requirements before your own is never something simple to do. Yet, to find genuine affection, you need to set your requirements aside for later once in a while.

**You're willing to leave for their advantage:**Adoring magnanimously doesn't imply that you stay come what may. There are times while adoring somebody implies that you need to leave to be magnanimous.If remaining is sitting idle yet causing what is happening or permitting codependency, then to be sacrificial, you have to stop the poisonous relationship you offer and know when it is simply time to leave, so they can develop, mend, and take care of themselves.

**You're glad to think twice about:**Being magnanimous doesn't generally imply that you need to totally surrender all that and consistently yield. At times, being sacrificial to seeing someone more about figuring out how to think twice about cooperating to ensure that you're both getting what you really want.

**You don't inquire whether it's not what they need:**Very much like a boomerang, at times we need to liberate things and check whether they return. It is not difficult to put a fit of remorse on somebody to make them stay or to make them reliant upon you with the goal that you don't lose them.In any case, magnanimous love at times implies that you need to set somebody free and make it acceptable for them to continue on the off chance that the relationship isn't mostly ideal for you both.

**You put your desire aside:**

In a relationship, you will have your singular objectives and your joined ones. There will be times when you could have to forfeit your needs to permit your accomplice to sparkle. Being sacrificial implies that you have to take the rearward sitting arrangement now and again to permit your accomplice to accomplish their fantasies and their maximum capacity.

There will be times in your future when you can work on you and spotlight on your way. Being caring means keeping an eye on everything occasionally so your accomplice can go tempest the palace.

**You have weighty shoulders:**Being magnanimous means setting yourself to the side, and assuming somebody needs you to have weighty shoulders, having them. Not being protective, or thinking about things too literally, magnanimous love implies that you identify with what your cherished one is going through, and you set your sentiments to the side to areas of strength to be they can't be.

**You don't pass judgment:**Judging is perhaps of the most exceedingly terrible human quality that we have. Being sacrificial in adoration implies that you don't decide what somebody is doing. That doesn't imply that you don't defy them when you think they are harming themselves, nor does it imply that you permit a terrible way of behaving to proceed.
It simply implies that you don't put judgment on why somebody is acting how they are, you assist with modifying the ways of behaving that hurt them in a non-critical manner.
**You tune in and don't make suppositions:**At the point when you are rehearsing caring affection, it intends that rather than making suppositions about why somebody is acting a specific way or doing what they are doing, you carve out an opportunity to pay attention to them.Standing by listening to someone else that you love when you would rather not hear it tends to be undeniably challenging. Tuning in without judgment is the best way to give benevolent love.

**You're glad to assume the best about them:**Being somebody's ally generally and giving genuine love is in some cases not exactly simple or easy.Regardless of whether they have given you down access in the past, benevolent love is about continuously assuming the best about them and accepting that they can adapt to the situation rather than setting up an unavoidable outcome and afterward pausing for a minute or two and saying "I knew it."

**Functioning collectively – There's no 'I' in group:**Benevolent love is tied in with being unified with somebody and not being out for your objectives. Cooperating is vital to benevolent love, and that implies that you're not self-serving or continuously attempting to get everything you could possibly want.

Cooperating is the foundation of sacrificial love.

**You change your arrangements since they need you more:**Surrendering things isn't mainly something simple to do. There are times when you could need to forego things that are vital in your life assuming somebody you love requires you more.

Having the option to put the requirements of another person above what is vital to you is caring and a phenomenal method for showing love.

**Not giving in because it's simpler:**
Love shows restraint, love is benevolent, and it additionally is difficult. Connections aren't straightforward. They are commonly when they out-and-out suck, as a matter of fact! Having the option to make it happen and go through the harsh spots is what's truly going on with benevolent love.

**Consuming the boat:**There is an old story about a skipper team to an abandoned new land, and when the group had left the boat, and everybody had dumped, they pivoted to track down the boat on fire.

The skipper had set it aflame, saying they all endure together, or they die alone. Consuming your boat implies that regardless, it is absolutely impossible that out of benevolent love. You simply need to figure it out and traverse it. Moreover, some of the time you feel like you can't hang on anymore, however you simply do.

**Saying "in disorder and in wellbeing" and the importance it:**At the point when you say "I do," or when you are in a serious relationship, there are times when things don't go precisely as expected. Since actually, there will come when we as a whole should leave the earth, one of you will go first.Or then again, misfortune sometimes strikes, and it could drive one of you to deal with the other. Rehearsing magnanimous love implies that when the other individual necessities you, whether this is a result of an intense disease or a drawn out inability, you will go the long stretch. Benevolent love could mean reclassifying all that you know and your jobs inside a relationship to make it work.

**Following through with something and anticipating nothing, consequently:**
Sacrificial love implies that you will give however much you get. It additionally implies that you don't play the "unfortunate me" card or cause the other to feel obliged when you truly do need to get the additional leeway.Benevolent love is rarely remorseful or angry. It implies you are continuously ready to give similarly however much you would expect, while perhaps not more, for and from the individual you love.

**You acknowledge them as they are, blemishes what not:**

No one is great, however sacrificial love pushes you to acknowledge an individual for what their identity is, without wanting to change them. You realize that they have blemishes, however you additionally acknowledge that you have them as well. It's practically similar to you love their defects as much as there in addition to focuses! An imperfect individual is a genuine individual, by the day's end.

**You don't hold hard feelings:**
Part of tolerating somebody for what their identity is additionally implies realizing that they will mess up incidentally. At the point when that occurs, you don't hold it against them, and you don't permit it to continue to spring up from here on out. When the statement of regret has been made, you let it proceed to gain from it together.

**You're willing to assist them with turning into all that they can be:**Assisting somebody with arriving at their true capacity and understanding their fantasy takes time and exertion. At times, we simply don't have that, and we're too centered around ourselves. Sacrificial love implies you're willing to assist somebody with being the absolute most ideal form of themselves, and that you're glad to contribute an opportunity to do as such.

## What is the distinction between benevolent love and self-centered love?

The two are frequently confounded or thought to be the same thing. There is an undeniable different between sacrificial love and narrow-minded love. You needn't bother with being a mind specialist to understand that caring is better compared to self-centered! Anyway, what is the distinction? Self-centered love doesn't feel as normal as sacrificial love. It's frequently constrained, or at times feels like it's only happening for a really long time. Maybe one or the two accomplices need to continue on, however don't have any desire to say it. Caring adoration is tolerating and free. It feels lighter and more harmonious.In some cases, there are difficult situations and contentions, however these are managed all the more effectively because the two accomplices are in total agreement.

If your relationship is continually brimming with show, a pattern of contentions, and feels debilitating, it's not caring. All things considered, one accomplice could be less contributed than the other, or just searching for an exit plan. At the point when your relationship is brimming with sacrificial love, you become together, and you're joyfully pushing the other one to be all that they can be.Does your relationship feel amicable more often than not, or does it seem like a consistent drama of the show? That is most likely the most ideal way to sort out whether it is magnanimous or childish love.

## Is caring affection actually that sound?

This is an inquiry that is posed to a ton. It's critical that your requirements are met similarly as much as your accomplice's, so is magnanimous love sound? The exceptionally straightforward response is, indeed, the same length as the two accomplices are adoring benevolently. If one accomplice is doing all the giving and the other is taking, it's a catastrophe waiting to happen.Nothing bad can really be said about putting someone before yourself for however long you're doing it for the right reasons. In a caring relationship, there will be times when you want additional help. All things considered, your accomplice will put your necessities before theirs. Then, while they're battling, you'll drop a couple of things that mean a lot to you for some time and show up for them.A compromise circumstance swings this way and that. You both have each other's wellbeing in heart and that is the reason it's not unfortunate. At the point when the relationship is loaded with two-sided caring adoration, you construct each other up and turn into an imposing power!

## Is your accomplice a childish sweetheart, while you're a caring darling?

Assuming your accomplice is doing any of the accompanying consistently, that focuses on self-centered love on their part:

1. Never there when you really want them, yet you're dependably close by when they're down.
2. Not one for expressions of remorse.
3. Never down to split the difference and consistently needs things their way.
4. Not especially intrigued assuming you're upset or feeling down.

5. Not steady of novel thoughts or amazing open doors that come your direction.
6. Continuously considering themselves before you.
For this situation, it doesn't make any difference assuming that you're dropping all that and being the steady accomplice, the relationship is out of equilibrium. Everybody merits benevolent love, regardless of whether it means holding up a short time to get it.Caring affection isn't something that generally falls into place without any issues. There are times when you need to give a higher amount of yourself than you could have at first figured you would. It implies setting yourself to the side sometimes and putting another person's necessities before yours and anticipating nothing consequently. For better or for more, terrible does at times really imply "in negative ways."

# CHAPTER 4

## The Excellence limits

You lock the entryway when you leave your condo, set a superb out-of-office message when you take some time off, and quite often express no to party solicitations that begin after 10 p.m. Yet, regarding your relationship, your limits are really nonexistent because, indeed, why is that heartfelt? At the point when the message is frequently to such an extent that genuine romance method being around your accomplice constantly and being willing to do anything for them, saying "no" can feel like a reason for a separation. However, it ends up, it is conceivable and is really a better way to deal with your relationship to show you care for your accomplice while as yet showing that you care for your time and values.Expressing our limits is tied in with recognizing ourselves and our necessities, our first, and most significant relationship is with ourselves. If we don't watch out for this relationship, we won't have the option to oversee ideal associations with others.

Regardless of the amount it seems like you and your accomplice could possibly guess every others' thoughts, imparting straightforwardly about your boundaries is in every case great. On the off chance that an accomplice is passed on to speculate about what they may be, they can over and over accomplish something you're not happy with, making you become increasingly more angry while they don't enroll their way of behaving is irritating you. Allow these sentiments to rot, and you're seeing possible adverse consequences on the quality, on the off chance that not the achievement, of the relationship. In any case, as in most things, there are solid and undesirable ways of beginning having these discussions. Here's the beginning and end, you really want to be familiar with how to define limits in a relationship.

## For what reason are limits significant for a solid relationship?

A great deal of times, when individuals hear "limits," they have pictures of a wall or one more hindrance that you set up among yourself and your accomplice. They're thought to be a negative part of a relationship, something that an accomplice uses to close you out. In any case, specialists say, nothing could be further from reality.Limits are approaches to guaranteeing both your and your accomplice's close to home prosperity. You can tell your accomplice precisely what you want out of the relationship and how you're willing to help them, while additionally encouraging that you will regard what they need and what they will do. Having this discussion right off the bat in a relationship assists with limiting clash, hatred, and tension pushing ahead. Everything unquestionably revolves around addressing your accomplice's requirements yet in addition esteeming your own.By defining limits, we are affirming that we accept that we deserve regard.

## Which limits don't work in a relationship?

It's a lot better to examine your needs, requirements, and assumptions before it arrives. Currently, somebody in the relationship reaches a stopping point and can't take a specific way of behaving any longer. The most horrendously horrible method for trying and put down a limit is the point at which you are doing as such at the time, and bitterly.Something critical to remember, when you understand something is a limit for you, you likewise get to save the ideal for that limit not to be totally inflexible. A decent limit is porous. You require limits that, occasionally, an individual can cross, whether they're physical or profound, yet you likewise don't maintain that they should be nonexistent. The key here is that you, not any other person get to choose when you need to twist a specific limit.Expressing something if a limit is likewise not a reason for controlling a way of behaving. An accomplice following your area, restricting what you can wear, or directing who you can see are activities that ought to provide you an opportunity to stop and think.

The most effective method to define limits in your relationship:

**Begin with self-reflection:**It's a good idea that on the off chance that you don't have the foggiest idea what your limits are, you will not have the option to impart them to your accomplice, really. While this could appear glaringly evident, many individuals don't understand that something is a limit until a specific way of behaving of their accomplices begins to irritate them.Before you can discuss limits with your accomplice, you need to truly understand what your limits are and now and again, individuals don't. You need to go through the mindfulness stage before you can truly speak with your accomplice.

**Try not to tarry:**On the off chance that you don't contemplate what your limits are, your accomplice will end up characterizing them for you likely, by crossing them (over and over). This is one of the primary motivations behind why, inevitably, individuals get angry toward their accomplices or genuinely regret themselves when they see they were not as clear about defining their limits.

## Consider: contact, words, time, and distance.

It's not generally simple to understand what your limits are, particularly in another relationship. I suggest contemplating your limits in four classes: contact, words, time, and physical and profound distance.

So perhaps you're just cool with handholding openly (contact), will not acknowledge ridiculing (words), esteem alone time (time), and care about moving gradually, inwardly, (seeing someone). Then, at that point, pay attention to your instinct, On the off chance that you're not prepared to move that limit, anybody who merits being with you will regard that.

**Recount your limits:**On the off chance that no doubt about it "limit setting," it might assist with reflecting on them in the mornings, perhaps related to a goal setting practice until they just become mostly you think and act. "At the point when you 'are' an individual with clear limits, you don't have to 'do' limit setting consistently." Very much like eating right and working out, it turns out to be simply one more piece of your way of life.

**Begin the limit setting conversation**: There's nobody method for discussing your limits. Perhaps conversations about, say, how you both feel about dropping plans could come up naturally, while others, similar to your need to give assent before your accomplice has a go at anything masochistic in the room, may should be expressed more proactively. One way into such discussions is to ask your accomplice first the way that they feel about specific lines. Is messaging during the working day cool or problematic? Is dropping a date effectively excusable or absolutely hostile? Sentiments on kissing openly? "It can feel fake since it's anything but a discussion we're accustomed to having, except if our limits have been disregarded," Yet it'll get more straightforward. After some time, it can feel more regular, and you make it your own.

**Show others how it's done:**It's adequately not to simply discuss your limits. You additionally need to carry on like somebody who merits regard. At the point when you profoundly regard yourself, it appears in specific ways of behaving. For example, is your accomplice generally served first at supper? Is it true that

you are mainly the one to change your timetable when there's a contention? "Know whether you are continually conveying messages that you come in second.
**Utilize a scale from 1 to 10 to get down on limit crossing.**
Once in a while, limits get crossed. It's the way you handle that infringement that can represent the deciding moment in a relationship. In the first place, try not to address the slip up seemingly out of the blue, and on second thought, raise your anxiety when you're both quiet. "On the off chance that the individual you are dating is dependably a couple of moments late and this irritates you, you want to talk about this merciful however solidly. Utilizing a size of 1 to 10 to clarify how significant each point is to you. Saying, "Ugh, it's so it, no doubt about it" possible won't bring about any massive changes to pester that. Saying, "On a scale from 1 to 10, speediness is an 8, that is that it means a lot to me" ought to get the job done.
**Use "I" explanations and other advisor supported discussion methods:**
Start the discussion by setting the stage, and that implies taking note of something that you

esteem in the relationship. You could open with, "You're vital to me, so I need to come clean with you," for instance. Then, name the conduct you might want to change utilizing "I" proclamations to make sense of how that activity (or inaction) not the individual, causes you to feel. Perhaps you say, "I feel baffled when you say you'll cover the bills, and afterward you don't send in the cash." At last, ask for the way of behaving to change. For example: "I believe that you should finish when you say you'll do.

**Perceive that uneasiness is typical and, here and there, socially implemented:** Being confident can feel awkward to some extent, since ladies are regularly associated with being more passive. Occasionally, we need to move past how we're mingled, not to shout out for our own sake. In any case, when you do, it will pay off. It very well may be truly liberating it's showing that you regard yourself, and it's showing the way in which you hope to be dealt with, it can truly make a great construction of a sound relationship.

**Know your issues:**Some limit infringement, as physical or psychological mistreatment, ought to be straight-up huge issues in all cases.

Others, similar to disloyalty, might be less obvious. One way or the other, assuming that you've followed these means and your accomplice keeps on disregarding your limits, accept that as a serious sign, this relationship isn't really for you. Your issues are major issues for an explanation, and if your accomplice doesn't regard them, that is as great an explanation as any to cut off the friendship before it becomes unfortunate.

# CHAPTER 5

## The most effective method to Cherish and Be Adored

A better approach to cherish and be adored is an elective way to deal with connections and profound associations that go past conventional standards and designs. It recognizes the variety and smoothness of human encounters, inclinations, and wants, and urges people to investigate and characterize their own extraordinary ways to cherish and satisfaction.Building serious areas of strength for a caring relationship requires exertion, responsibility, and a comprehension of what it means to genuinely cherish and be adored. Establishing a cherishing and supporting climate for both you and your accomplice permits your relationship to prosper and develop.

## The most effective method to Cherish Your Accomplice the Manner in which They Need to Be Adored

As much as being enamored can feel like a characteristic state we either experience or don't, we have a significantly surprisingly say in it. Research has demonstrated the way that making additional caring moves can cause couples to feel more enamored. Along these lines, there's a lot of truth to the idea that adoration is more an action word than a thing.The more we express love, the more we touch off it in our accomplice and develop it in ourselves.Pondering the manners in which we show love can be a strong practice for keeping our sentiments fit as a fiddle in a relationship. The vital isn't to exclusively zero in on our sensations of fondness, however to contemplate what our accomplice sees as adoration. As such, what explicit activities could that particular individual experience as cherishing? It's a typical and reasonably instinctual thing to give love in the manner we would feel it. For certain individuals, that implies giving their accomplice cards and gifts, communicating heaps of fondness, and much of the time saying "I love you." For other people, love is something all the more relaxed, a peaceful enthusiasm for the other individual wherein you give them space to do whatever they might feel like doing.A ton of issues in connections can focus on misconceptions or miscommunications about the things that cause every individual to feel cherished. For example, one individual might anticipate that their accomplice should know instinctually what they need and need. They might feel hurt by their accomplice when they unavoidably fail to understand the situation, thinking things like, "I would do this for them. Is there any good reason why they wouldn't do that for me?" The response might be that their accomplice simply doesn't consider that specific activity to be significant or helpful, similarly. They basically have various things they classify as articulations of adoration.

For instance, a couple I worked with frequently got into warmed contentions around their commemoration. For one accomplice, the day made a big difference to her, and she needed to celebrate by accomplishing something together. She considered the event a reason to let her significant other knows how she had an outlook on him and what she cherished about their relationship. She jumped at the chance to design escapes and heartfelt meals, and was in numerous instances frustrated that her significant other didn't invest a similar energy into celebrating.

For her, significant other, the actual date didn't hold as much importance. While he frequently got her a little gift or roses for their commemoration, he didn't see the point in making any one day such no joking matter. He felt like what made the most considerable difference was that he valued his significant other and their relationship consistently. Sentiment, he accepted, ought to be more unconstrained and can't exactly be arranged. Their two viewpoints definitely left one of them disheartened. While she was feeling hurt and dismissed, he was feeling forced and ignored. What at last assisted them with arriving at a comprehension was every one of them getting some margin to imagine the other's perspective and perceive that the things that caused their accomplice to feel cherished and appreciated were not the same as their own.When they embraced that basic situation, they had the option to consider their activities to be essential for an objective to cause the other individual to feel esteemed rather than a penance that bowed them rusty. Since every one of them held the longing to make the other cheerful, they had the option to be more open about how that affected their accomplice. Notwithstanding, it took them to understand that affection itself reduced to atrocities in comparison to they envisioned.For the spouse, he understood that sort and recognizing words, expressions of warmth, and motions amounted to a lot more to his significant apart from gifts that weren't as private. For the spouse, she began to comprehend the amount it intended to her better half to allow things to happen normally. She had the option to allow their commemoration to unfurl all the more precipitously and not put as much tension on only one single day of festivity. All things considered, she could see the value in the caring ways her accomplice was over time. There is a wide range of variables that figure out what every one of us encounters as adoration, from our connection examples to our essential nature. However, being interested and open to our accomplice's exceptional approach to feeling cherished can make us a superior, more adjusted accomplice. Anyway, how might we "improve" at understanding what our accomplice needs and needs?

**Pay attention to what they're talking about.** At the point when we invest a great deal of energy with somebody, from one perspective, we might feel we realize them much improved than any other individual. Then again, we might quit seeing specific things about them as they become more natural to us. This isn't because we're not intrigued or couldn't care less. It's frequently because our lives can get going, routinized, or agreeable so that we stop effectively getting to know the other individual.Focusing on what our accomplice says seems like the clearest guidance we'll at any point hear, however, it's something we need to remind ourselves to continue to do. Give careful consideration to when they notice something that is important to them or something that invigorates them. Urge them to be vocal about and request what they need.

## Focus on how they express their sentiments.

As well as hearing what they express, we ought to constantly attempt to see what illuminates our accomplice. It's simple to recognize the times when they appear to be exhausted and continue to actually take a look at their telephones from those where they're grinning and enlivened. This doesn't mean we're liable for fulfilling them 100% of the time. It's simply an approach to being adjusted and delicate to what causes them to wake up and to feel most themselves. This mindfulness assists us with really knowing our accomplices and comprehending the sorts of things that cause them to feel seen and cherished.

## Check in with your accomplice (and yourself)

Not a solitary one of us are telepaths, and we can't be anticipated to intuit what someone else needs and needs consistently. It's more than alright to get clarification on some pressing issues and urge our accomplice to tell us where they're at and what they require from us. By that equivalent measure, we ought to continue to check in with ourselves about what we want and need to cause us to feel cherished and satisfied. However, much as could reasonably be expected, we ought to open up to our accomplice about these things – not anticipating that they should mind read by the same token. By empowering a free and normal to and fro, we become more defenseless against one another and more equipped for offering each other what we truly care about.

**Notice how they express love.**
Chances are, the warm ways our accomplice treats us are to some degree intelligent of a way they appreciate being dealt with. On the off chance that they search out a great deal of actual contact or enjoy little demonstrations of liberality and benevolence, they might partake in something very similar to us. Obviously, this doesn't need to be taken in a real sense, and no errand should be matched precisely. For instance, it's entirely normal for every individual to carry specific extraordinary things to the

relationship. One accomplice might just appreciate doing the other's clothing, since it fulfills them, while the other lean towards enormous, clearing heartfelt signals. The point here doesn't imply that we shouldn't have our singular approaches to being wanting to one another. Rather, it's simply one more way we can be careful and receptive to specific activities that could cause our accomplice to feel recognized.

**Acknowledge your accomplice's necessities as unique in relation to your own.**
Connections ought not be about penance. On the off chance that fulfilling someone else on a reliable premise implies making ourselves hopeless, something may truly be off, and the relationship might worth looking at. Nonetheless, we ought to constantly be embracing of the way that our accomplice is a different individual from ourselves. While making each other blissful can be our very own enormous piece of joy, every one of our sentiments exists separate from the other's.

This is all to say that it's acceptable for you to need more friendship and for your accomplice to need more correspondence. It's acceptable for one individual to feel more cherished by their accomplice cleaning the counter than saying "I love you." Others could require the words. We each have various things to offer that would be useful and propose to one another. It's excessive for every one of our longings to adjust precisely consistently to partake in an equivalent and cherishing relationship. The only thing that is important is that every one of us keeps an open progression of interest, inventiveness, and energy around communicating our affection to somebody we helpfully as of now love. Couples who constantly look at and characterize how love affects every one of them have the most obvious opportunity in regard to keeping that feeling invigorated, both in their accomplice and in themselves.

## The most effective method to Love and be Cherished

To be cherished seeing someone, it is fundamental to develop and sustain a profound association with your accomplice. Love isn't something that works out more or less by accident yet is a consequence of persistent endeavors, understanding, and shared regard. On the off chance that you wish to be cherished seeing someone, are a few critical viewpoints to zero in on:

**Open Correspondence:** Correspondence is the core of any solid relationship. Lay out a culture of transparent correspondence with your accomplice. Offer your viewpoints, sentiments, and wants merciful and really, and listen effectively to your accomplice. Really try to grasp their perspective and approve their feelings. By cultivating successful correspondence, you make a completely safe space that empowers close to home closeness.

**Show Appreciation:** Cause your accomplice to feel esteemed and appreciated. Offer thanks for the easily overlooked details they accomplish for yourself and recognize their endeavors.

Little signals like saying "Thank you," leaving an adoration note, or commending them truly can go far in causing them to feel cherished and esteemed.

**Quality Time:** Commit quality chance to enjoy with your accomplice and focus on their presence in your life. Participate in exercises that you both appreciate to make shared encounters and recollections. Set to the side interruptions and spotlight on your accomplice earnestly. Exhibiting that you truly appreciate their conversation will cause them to feel exceptional and adored.

**Backing and Support:** Show up for your accomplice through various challenges. Offer your help and consolation in their interests, dreams, and objectives. Approve their yearnings and give a place of refuge to them to communicate their weaknesses. Show sympathy and assist them with exploring life's difficulties. By being their team promoter, you encourage a cherishing and sustaining climate.

**Trust and Genuineness:** Trust is the groundwork of a caring relationship. Tell the truth and straightforward with your accomplice, developing a climate of dependability and unwavering quality. Keep away from misleading or concealing data, as it can dissolve trust after some time. Trust is worked through steady activities and words that line up with respectability and genuineness.

**Close to home Accessibility:** Be genuinely present for your accomplice. Offer them a place of refuge to share their feelings, fears, and nerves. Practice undivided attention, compassion, and understanding establishing a steady climate. By being genuinely accessible, you become their stone, offering solace and a feeling of safety.

**Self-improvement:** Put resources into your self-improvement, both exclusively and as a couple. Develop your inclinations, work on personal growth, and urge your accomplice to do likewise. By ceaselessly advancing, you expand the relationship and motivate development in your accomplice too.

**Closeness and Fondness:** Actual touch, closeness, and friendship are fundamental parts of feeling cherished. Show your accomplice love through embraces, kisses, clasping hands, and spending personal minutes together. Moreover, keep a solid sexual association, as it can develop the close to home bond and increment sensations of affection and fascination.

**Tolerance and Split the difference:** Connections aren't generally going great, and clashes are inescapable. Practice tolerance and look for understanding during testing times. Approve your accomplice's feelings and perspective, and split the difference for the relationship. By showing adaptability and understanding, you exhibit your obligation to the relationship and your accomplice's bliss.

**Shock Motions:** Incidentally, you collaborate with signals that show your affection and appreciation. Plan an insightful night out, set up their #1 feast, or give them a little gift that mirrors their inclinations. These shocks can reignite the flash in your relationship and cause your accomplice to feel unquestionably cherished and esteemed.Keep in mind, love is a constant cycle that requires exertion, understanding, and magnanimity. By encapsulating these characteristics and reliably exhibiting your adoration for your accomplice, you can develop a profound and enduring adoration in your relationship.

# CHAPTER 6

## The baffling change force of adoration

Love is a strong power that can change and rise above the constraints of human connections. It can transform enemies into companions, recuperate wounds, and achieve significant self-improvement and change. The strange change force of adoration in a relationship is for sure a wonder to see.One of the most surprising parts of adoration's groundbreaking power is its capacity to disintegrate hostility and develop kinship. At the point when love enters a relationship, it can relax hearts and eliminate the hindrances that different people. Love can transform adversaries into partners and make understanding and sympathy where just antagonism existed. This change can significantly affect the two people included, permitting them to develop and advance in manners they never imagined.Love additionally can recuperate wounds and retouch broken hearts. Connections are not resistant to difficulties and clashes, and it is at these times that the groundbreaking force of adoration genuinely sparkles. Love can achieve absolution and advance recuperating, permitting people to push ahead and revamp their trust and association. It can repair profound scars and make a safe and supporting space for development and recuperating.

Moreover, love can light self-improvement and change. At the point when people experience love in a relationship, they frequently end up roused to turn out to be better renditions of themselves. Love can motivate people to defy their apprehensions, break liberated from old examples and propensities, and take a stab at individual and shared development. It provokes people to turn out to be more mindful, compassionate, and able to think twice about. The groundbreaking force of adoration in such a manner encourages self-awareness and prompts a seriously satisfying and significant life.Love likewise can change our view of our general surroundings. At the point when we are enamored, we will regularly see the magnificence in all things and everybody. Love opens our hearts and psyches, permitting us to see past the surface and interface with the more profound quintessence of others. It makes an air of inspiration and confidence, changing our standpoint and improving our general prosperity. This groundbreaking force of affection empowers us to encounter life all the more completely and find delight in even the least difficult of things.In any case, it is critical to take note of that the groundbreaking force of adoration can happen in sound and adjusted connections. Love can't independently fix poisonous elements or tackle well established issues. It requires open correspondence, shared regard, and an eagerness to deal with difficulties together. Love can guide and support change. However, it is eventually up to the people required to participate in the process effectively.

Let's dive into the different aspects of the secretive change force of affection in connections.
**Close to home Reverberation:** Love makes a profound reverberation between two

individuals. It can transform customary minutes into exceptional ones. Straightforward motions and shared encounters take on new importance and significance when love is available. The profound bond that adoration structures can change people by giving a feeling of safety, having a place, and reason.

**Self-Revelation:** Love frequently fills in as a mirror, mirroring one's actual self back to them. Regarding a caring relationship, people might be urged to defy their feelings of trepidation, instabilities, and weaknesses. This course of self-revelation can be both testing and extraordinary, prompting self-improvement and personal growth.

**Sympathy and Understanding:** Love has the noteworthy capacity to cultivate compassion and understanding. At the point when you genuinely love somebody, you become sensitive to their necessities, wants, and sentiments. This elevated sympathy can prompt critical individual changes, as you figure out how to consider and focus on the prosperity of your accomplice, frequently harming your longings.

**Persistence and Resilience:** Love can test one's understanding and resistance in different ways. It provokes people to adjust and acknowledge the defects and idiosyncrasies of their accomplices. This interaction can prompt an exceptional change, as individuals figure out how to be more persistent, excusing, and understanding.

**Inspiration and Desire:** Love can be a strong inspiration. It motivates people to work harder, defeat obstructions, and take a stab at a superior future, for themselves as well as for their friends and family. The longing to give and mind to one's accomplice and family can drive people to accomplish things they may likely have never imagined.

**Mending and Versatility:** Love can recuperate profound injuries and upgrade strength. In the midst of trouble, a caring relationship can give a place of refuge to people to discuss their thoughts and track down comfort. This recuperating and backing can prompt close to home development and newly discovered strength.

**Shared Objectives and Yearnings:** Love frequently prompts the development of shared objectives and goals. At the point when two individuals in a relationship meet to seek after normal goals, they can encounter a wonderful change, as they figure out how to team up, split the difference, and accomplish together.

**Profound Development:** Certain individuals find that adoration has an otherworldly aspect. It tends to be viewed as a power that rises above the physical and profound, interfacing people on a more profound, deep level. This otherworldly part of adoration can prompt significant individual and close to home changes.

**Extraordinary Difficulties:** Love isn't generally going great; it can include difficulties and clashes. These hardships can be groundbreaking in themselves. They can compel people to face their weaknesses, convey all the more, and figure out how to think twice about adjusting.

All in all, the secretive change force of adoration in a relationship is certain. It can disintegrate aggression and develop companionship, mend wounds, light self-awareness, and change our view of the world. Love can draw out the best in us and lead us towards a really satisfying and significant association with others. Embracing this extraordinary force of adoration in our connections can genuinely be a life-changing encounter.

# CONCLUSION

Developing care inside the setting of connections is a significant and groundbreaking excursion that can prompt further associations, expanded capacity to understand people on a deeper level, and improved generally speaking prosperity. Care in connections involves the conscious and non-critical consideration regarding our own contemplations, sentiments, and ways of behaving, as well as those of our accomplices. It enables us to break liberated from responsive examples, encouraging more noteworthy comprehension and sympathy. By being available and completely took part in our collaborations, we can convey all the more really, resolve clashes with sympathy, and support a feeling that everything is safe and secure and confide in our connections.

In addition, the act of care assists us with rising above self image driven wants and connections, empowering us to embrace fleetingness and change with beauty. In doing as such, we can lessen enduring, as we figure out how to relinquish ridiculous assumptions and cultivate satisfaction with what is, as opposed to what we wish it to be. This internal change has the ability to swell outward, making a positive effect on our connections, making them stronger and amicable.

Generally, care in connections is an encouragement to set out on a significant excursion of self-revelation and association. It outfits us with the apparatuses to break liberated from the restrictions of our molded reactions, permitting us to encounter love, sympathy, and closeness in their most flawless and most certified structures. By focusing on this way, we can make more significant and persevering through bonds with others and, thus, track down satisfaction and bliss in the mind boggling woven artwork of our interconnected lives.

# MINDFULLY ATTACHED